""How to lose 70 LB in 3 months""

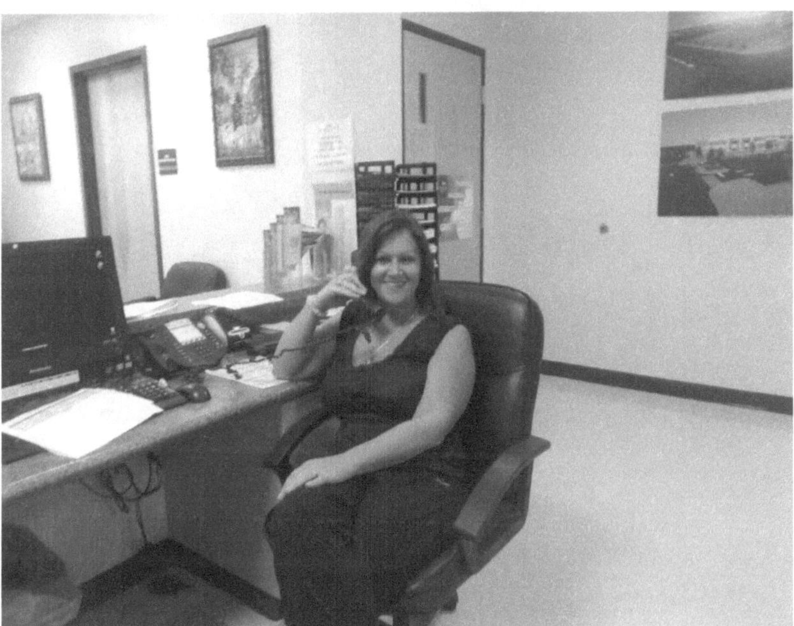

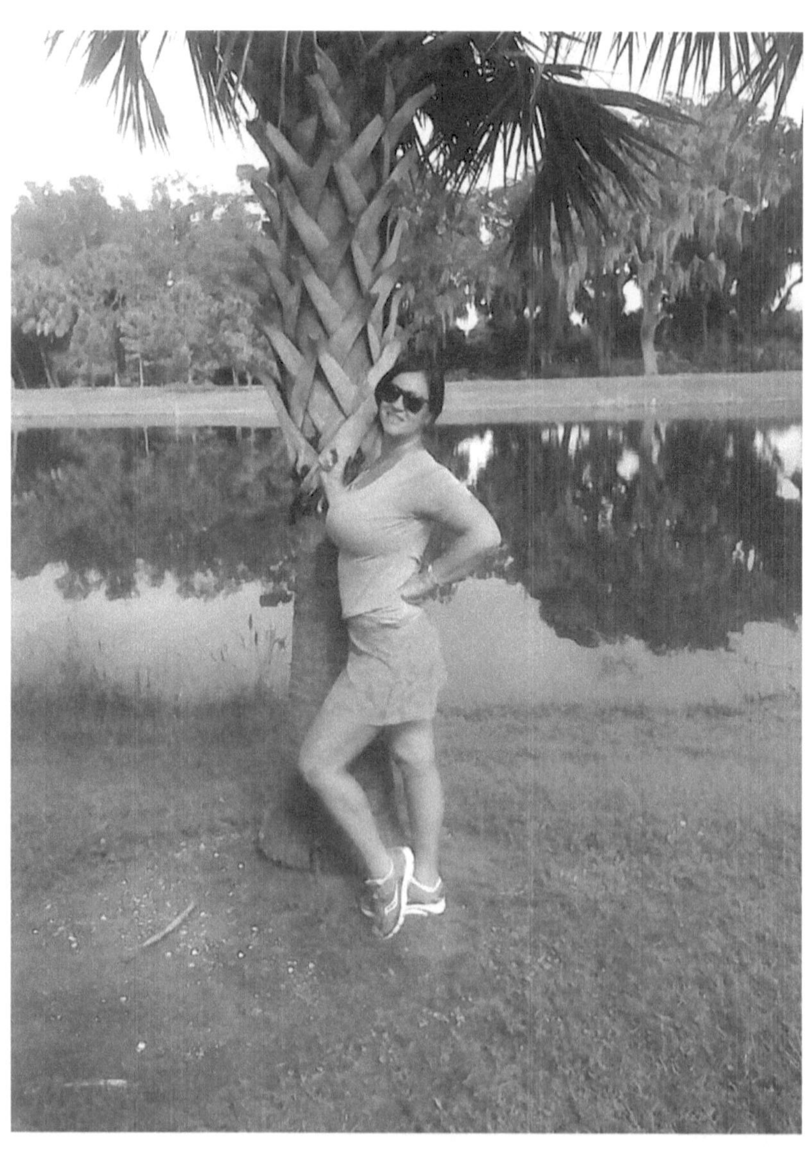

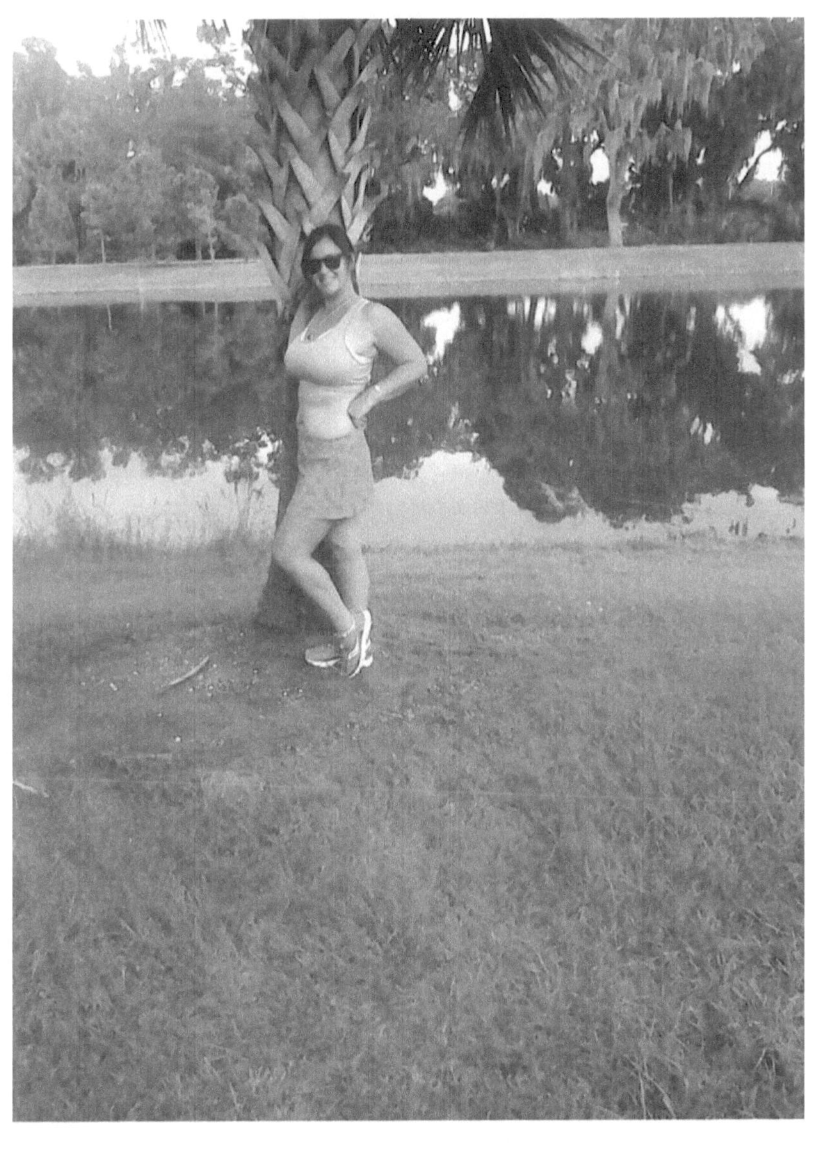

Preface:

This book is a guide and a few weigh loss tips on my weight loss journey, it content different stories, techniques and ideas you might find helpful in your weight loss try out, exercises, advises on keeping a food journal, I used motivation quotes, I hope I can inspire you to lose the weight you need to lose and fast! Happy reading, and weight droping! By Author : Vanessa Bush

Introduction:

"" How to lose 70 LB in 3 month"" Introduction: ----Lose Weight Fast by keeping a weight journal by your side for starter: Are you one of the many people who feel frustrated because you think you eat well and exercise regularly, but you just can't seem to lose weight? If so, a food journal is a great tool to help you reach your weight loss goals. It will help to determine any patterns in your eating habits, it will force you to be accountable for what you eat, and it will help you to see where you are consuming your "hidden" calories. The first thing I always tell people when they start to keep a food journal is to write down EVERY bite they put in their mouths. When most people think back over their day and what they had to eat, they go straight to their meals. It's amazing, though, how all of those calories you consume in between meals add up. You might think that one little piece of chocolate doesn't count, so you don't need to write it down, but that one little piece of chocolate every afternoon can add up to quite a few calories over the course of a week. Many mothers of young children tend to finish what their kids leave on their plates, but a chicken nugget here and three bites of macaroni and cheese there really add up! Be sure to write it down right after you eat so you don't forget. It's also important to be very specific when recording what you eat. For example, don't just write "roast beef sandwich" for lunch. Instead, write down "4 ounces turkey breast and 1 slice provolone cheese on wheat, with mustard, tomato and lettuce." The mayonnaise on your sandwich, butter on your baked potato, and creamer in your coffee may be contributing empty calories and fat to your diet that are easy to cut. And speaking of that coffee, don't forget to write down what you drink. Your mid-morning mocha latte or your glass of wine with dinner contain calories, too! Another thing to include in your food journal is the time you eat each meal or snack. Then, when you look back over your notes you can determine if you have any "trouble times." If you tend to eat junk every day around 4:00, then you might want to start having a healthy snack each day before that time, before you get too hungry and grab whatever is in sight. Or, if you see that you get the munchies every night while watching TV, you are probably eating out of boredom. When you know that is a problem for you, it's easier to distract yourself. Keeping a food journal can make you accountable for what you eat. I know that I am much less likely to have a big piece of cheesecake if I know I have to write it down! It will also make it much easier for you to determine what your eating patterns are and where you can cut calories that will make all the difference in your weight loss!

Summary of this book:

Introduction:

Chapter 1) Let me share with you my weight troubles...

Chapter 2) How I felt bigger than everyone!

Chapter 3) I starved myself!

Chapter 4) Make it happen now! Lets lose those extra pounds!

Chapter 5) Lose the weight and look beautiful!

Chapter 1)

let me share my secret with you;

I have spent my lifetime trying to lose weight it started when i was 13 the first time I noticed I was a little thicker and bigger than the rest of my class and in France this average size is small so being a medium-large will make you a fat person for sure. I remember guys laughing at me at the swimming pool or other making remarks about my weight when it was time to weight in during our annual nurse check up i was so afrais that I will find every escuse in the book to be escuse but it didnt always work I was afraid someone will her my weight and I will be the laughing stock for a other year but when I got on the scale that year the nurse say that my weight was proportionate to my muscle and bone mass and that I appear much thinner in person that what the scale actually say so it was some kind of compliment and I realize that the rest of the family was brought up with thick bones and has long has I was heaqlthy and sportive nothing lse should matter but even with this 3 to 4 sport I attended weekly I still struggle fitting in my tiny pants, my sexy shirt for the week-ends or invited party, I would hide under my taos until I could drop really quick ont he side bars by the swimming pool, I will never get on anyone's knees, too afraid someone might complain on how much I weight, basically, I was the 3rd fatty in an average class but never the biggest girl or guy. I felt bad for them but I couldn't imagine being that big and enduring this insult days on out, day after days, class after class, endurance classes was always the most humiliating for them they will break a tear and hide in the restroom.

Chapter 2) How I felt being too big;

I managed to keep my tone and muscle in shape so even if I was on the thick side I was energetic, very sportive and nothing like a fatty. what I struggle the most with was my chest it was always out of the norm, too big, too large too extreme, it felt like a huge handicap in my day to day chores and when the summer was in the corner I would spend hours trying to find a bathing suit who could make my breast look small and it never works.

Most guys were attracted like magnets and woman would always ask me" What is it like to have big breast?" I was like a weird thing to them but when you know people you not a thing anymore you a good friend and a person! So it really resumes to adolescence and complexity in its outrageous decay.

I am for equal rights in terms of big, large, tall, too small, too differents, too innadequate etc... but you can't feed a bull what it cannot see therefore we all accept one a other in different ways and by the way how fun would it be if we couldn't stir a hilarious laugh with anyone about others once in while that's what teenage years are about but trying to fit into a format has consequences and will affect your future so be careful how you see or want to see yourself in the future. You have to fit in sure but you can without any pain or humiliation. I was a popular one so I rarely endure humilation in my youth but just a few time in middle school when a crazy controling woman taugh I cheated with her boyfriend of 3 years who turn out to had cheat on her for over a decade without her knowing it but too make me pay for a crime I didnt commit, she stuck me in the bathroom after recess and lock me in the toilett and threat to burn my hands and smoke while breathing in my face and pulling my hair, i was terrorized and told a few friends of her behaviors but she was well known to have a great reputation of dangerous bitch so noone would want to confront her and some night she will follow me and take her knife out and get close to me and play with it near my body so I will freeze of fear, that was the night I was tearing in the bus and all my best friends cheared me up! Very traumatizing when a crazy weirdo wants revenge. lucky me I knew many people and had many friends so her bullshit didn't last forever until 2 years later she realized i knew many of her friends and didn't want to find out so she came to me and pretended to be sorry. I was obsessed with losing weight I hated to be bigger than most of my girlfriends that all could fit size 2 to 6 and I was fitting a size 8 to 9 to sometimes 10 and that was very large to them and it actually the size of shirt I needed to buy. In France, a size medium in America is a size extra large in France.

Chapter 3) I starve myself;

 I sometimes starve and starting to make myself throw up, once it started to work I decided to go dance more in clubs to lose some more and try every single weight loss pills on the market and diet programs, weight loss doctors, but I was a yo-yo maybe it was the pressure, maybe the stress, maybe these hormones, I was getting pimples all over my forehead and getting fatter, I remember being so disgusted staring at the scale. I spend the all year apprehending to find new ways to be dismissed from a field trip to swimming pools and when I got there I was shocked to hear that I actually wasn't so fat that was the first time from since I was 12 that I ever heard a guy said that I had a nice body! I was so happy that day, I dream to the day I wouldn't be called that anymore, party after party's date after date I was referred has the thick girls with enormous breast! and I wasn't a person sometimes I was just a breast nest to be hunted by stupid guys who will block my way to the hallways to either molest me or lift my shirt up, I was violated all the time and I talked about it to my closest friend but never really saw any dramatic trauma into it, just some lurcky looser wanting to annoy me, after I was called a monster for 1 year when I was 13 to 14 this was my worse year, it was either monster of pamela anderson or lolo ferrary during running activities. I love the winter because I could find comfort in so many beautiful sweater, pure silk, lycra or warm material and never have to worry about showing any fat. When I reach 16 we schedule a visit to get a breast reduction at a surgeon and after I listen to him and over analyze my option he gave me 2 years to make a decision because he figured I hadn't mature enough to really know what is best for me so guess what? for has long has I knew I wanted my breast gone forever but when I reach 18 I realized that I didn't want to carry scars and that if I was meant to be this way so be it and I could always work on losing weight. I wasn't so concerned anymore and I learned to leave with it so I was actually starting to realize that having tiny or small breast wasn't that great either and I was blessed. When I truly got thinner and started like a fit pretty woman I was on the top of the world and felt beautiful. At 17 my weight loss trouble stops and i promise myself that I will never be fat again and I never broke my promise at 19 I told myself that I will stop trying out hair colors because I realized that I had really had my natural hair color and I keep getting hair cut so I said: when I reach 20 I will have long beautiful hair: And so I did! I had locks, golden blonds long voluptuous hair and a great body I never needed to be on diet ever again my brain was hired on my diet and I will conform to it and it's only after a few years later when I heard people talking about pregnancy and getting so angry and eating like pigs that I realize how horrifying it would be for me if I overeat I will be a fatty again! I really didn't worry about it too much I knew how easily I could drop the weight and I won't overeat so problem fix! During occasion and celebration, those were this only times I will allow myself any fat or sugar so it was pretty easy to go shopping: No chocolate, No ice cream, no cookies, nothing containing any sugar beside fruits and sugar-free yogurts, no fat, no milk, only natural sugar, rarely I ll allow a few piece of dark chocolate and ice cream in the summer. I love food but I wasn't going to give in to change into a fat ballon for the sake of candies and chocolate bars. I was content, healthy and very energetic, I walked miles and miles like the type of Chinese woman you will see carrying her clothes basket over her head going to do laundry in the forest river and needed to walk 10 miles to get to it. I saw myself has the ruler of the valley, an explorer of nature, I love walking and I surely walk everywhere, my speed will increase and my discovery will never end even if I couldn't retain the names of every single flower, hermits, insects, plants etc.... I was like a car with no wheels. I spent so much time walking I figured I ll earn a medal of some kind but all I got was the pain in my hips and vicious people haunting me!!!! hahaha! I encounter too many crips on my walking trips and now I limit myself to only safe walking trails or beach walk if I am alone. SO!; To get back to my story I never realize I was on a strict diet all other those years from age 18 until 28 that I didn't crave anything in particular but I also was missing out on the greatest meals and never truly picked what I wanted in restaurant and buffets. So thats' when I figure that when I find out I was pregant I will take advantage of this opportunity to feed the baby to eat whathever I wanted but i never figured that I would overeat to the point of gaining 40lb in the 1st trimester and even know I was feeling so delighted and enjoying motherhood that when the doctor female announce in a very rude and offensive way announce that I was an obese overweight subject and needed to watch my weight....?? I looked at here like: "" Look at you little stick!! Just because you so skinny and probably have an anorexic disorder doesn't mean I am a fat woman! "" So I literally saw absolutely nothing wrong with my weight gain and everything wrong with her comments. when I reach my 9 month and after delivery, I had gained a total of 60lb!And that's when my life with the psychopath (My son's Dad) started when I was laying in bed trying to catch a breath, to learn to breastfeed, to sleep and having to do all of this while he would scream, yell, complain and eat all the food. I knew that eventually, I would need to lose weight but my focus was only on my new baby born, so a year later I did lose the weight on my own by walking and laying off fast food but after a few trauma and abuse and life and death experience I regained and reach my highest weight of 220lb that's when I became the " The Fat Girl" I need to loose the weight again, Look at me!!! It's so easy to gain but so hard to lose, you don't care what you look like when you in a survival mode fighting for an honorable cause against despicable dangerous people who can't get enough of your good nature. While I went from 165 to 220 in 2 months just by being behind a wheel and having to eat whatever I could afford so its a certainty that it wasn't healthy food but mainly the weight settled in from being cloture too many hours in my car and having just a few hours of walking each day. It's so weird because while I'm saving my son from those sick people having to stay at filthy woman shelters for a month who can be literally more damaging than actually healing you but it gave you a shelter but it's a nut house there and staying too long will make you go crazy. I met some case of very deranged people with vicious and manipulating ways even the volunteer and staff aren't very helpful but I kept 2 good influences of my wonderful stay and lean on the positive by seclusion. When my time was up I went on the road and couldn't care less how much I weight as long as I could remain safe that all that matters. It's only after settling down that I started to notice the weight gain. Here a few examples: Seeing your reflect in a miror or any type of reflexion material, seeing yourself in bad pictures and you get horrify!, looking at your rear miror and seeing a double chin that you didn't know existed, getting extreme pinching pain each time you sat too long on a chair, not walking straight because you feel so damn heavy, having to wear a lot of make up to hide the weight on your face, never being able to wear nice looking dresses and shirt because it will reveal your stomach fat. Nobody will ever open the door for you or flirt with you because you look like someone who let herself go. So here we are.... How did I lose 70lb in 90 days? I will share my secret with you and that is just me and if you want more detail go ahead and email me a question: kellybush@live.com My brother challenge me to lose 50 lb in 3 months, He could see how depress I look! I knew I needed a push so he offer to gave me $200 if i lost the weight. I usually rarely needed a push in the "How to get motivated" to get started, Starting point is usually this hardest part of the challenge... I did needed thoses "" Extra PUSHES"" pushed, everyone needs to get motivated once in a while, don't feel bad about it its totally normal, in our outermost desesperation and losses we can't find strength to get up and get moving and here what happen" He bet me $200 if I was to loose at least 50 lb in 3 months and at that time I couldn't even breath without anxiety, I couldn't walk without stress, I couldn't sleep without nightmare, I couldn't run for a minute. ""I took on the challenge"" (I knew I couldn't stay this way, I couldn't fit any clothes, I look like a whale, I feel ugly and heavy all the time, I sweat too much, I feel pain on my back all the time, its so demoralising and drowning to leave this way so I decide to get rid of this extra weight who was running my physical appearance and confidence.

16 Top Diet Plans That Are Actually Worth Trying

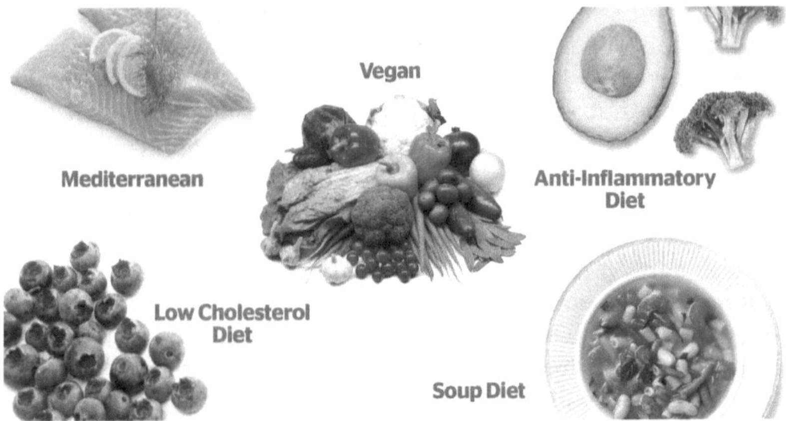

Fun fact: As soon as January rolls around, women are bombarded on the TV or Internet with diet messages every three seconds. In January last year, the word "diet" was used nearly 870,000 times across social media channels, according to an audit performed by Lean Cuisine. That's a lot. Thirty-eight percent of people have health and weight loss goals in January and they're ready to try something new — so long as it works. But there's one key thing to remember: There is no one-diet-fits-all plan (though that would make things easy). You have to find one that fits your lifestyle so you actually stick to it. With that in mind, here are the top diet plans that actually get results. All you have to do is pick one...and grab a fork.

Atkins

Paleo

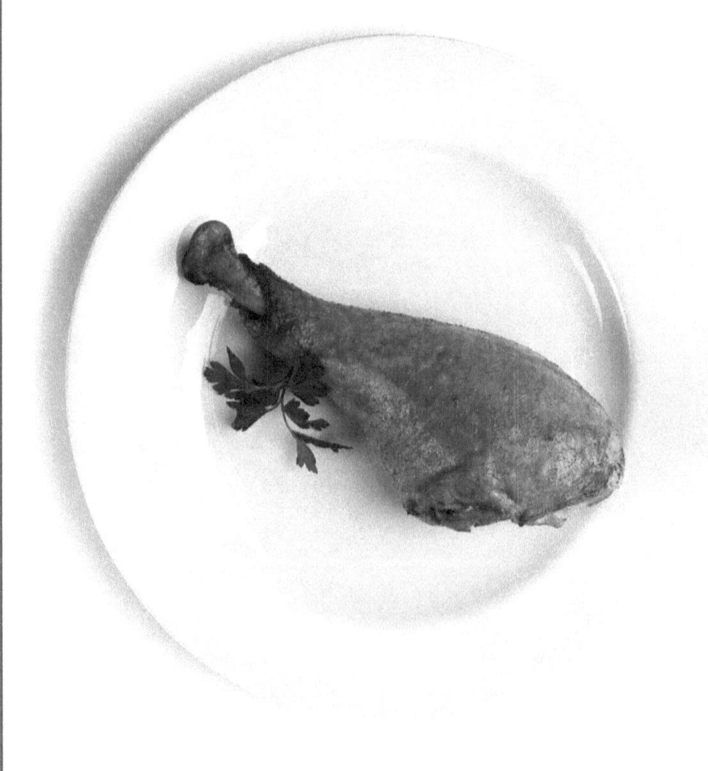

Mediterranean

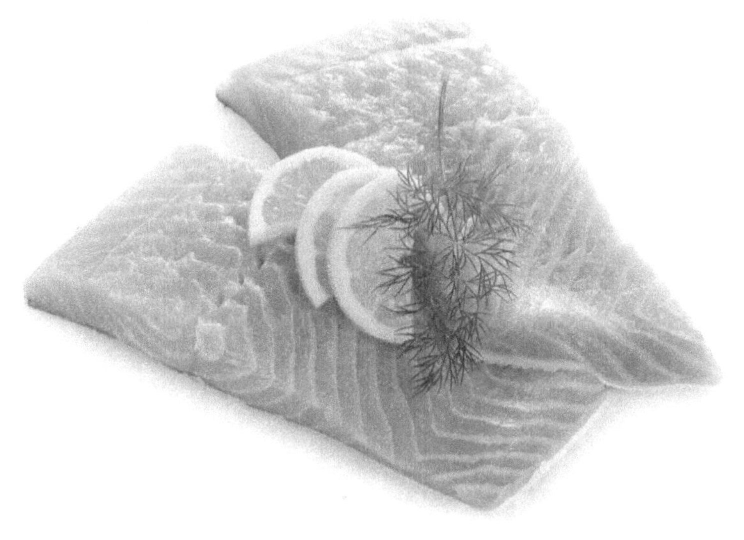

DASH

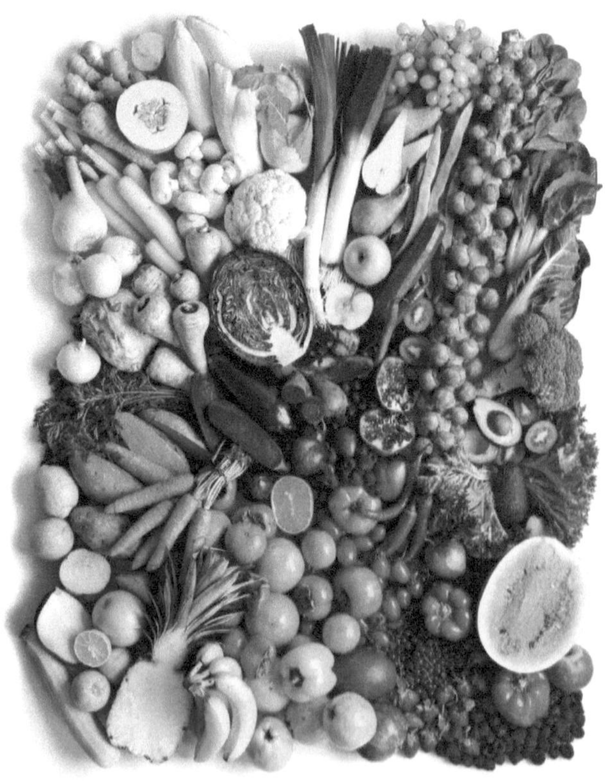

Vegan

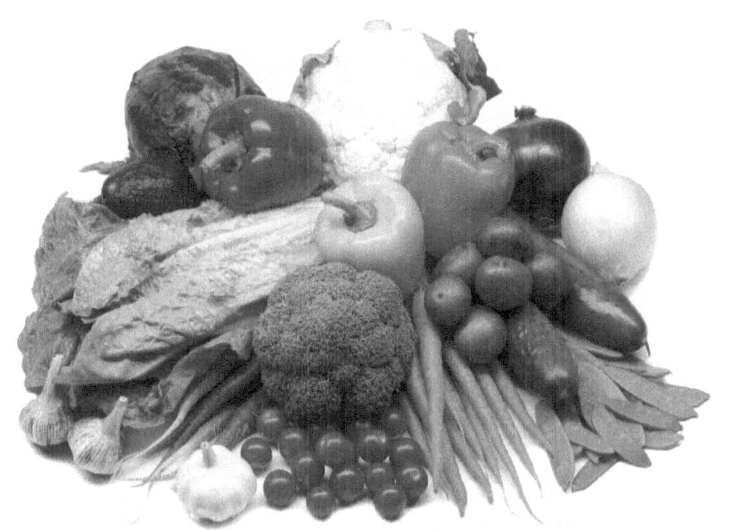

Vegetarian

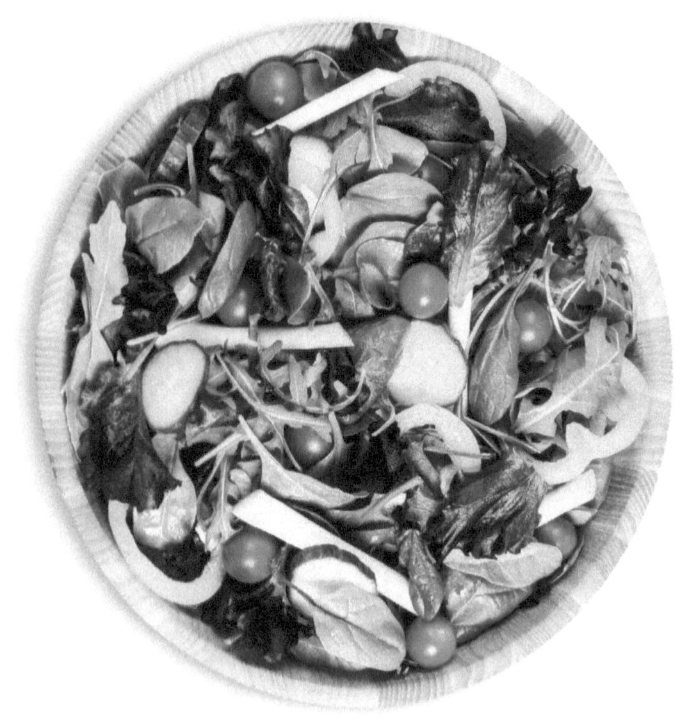

Nutrisystem

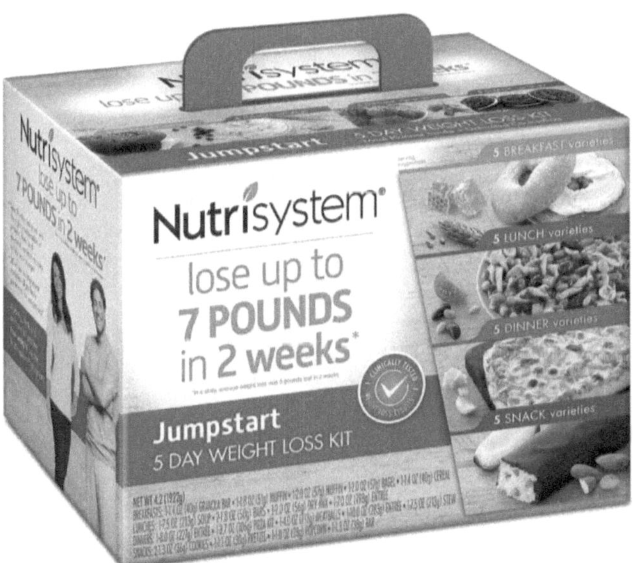

Jenny Craig

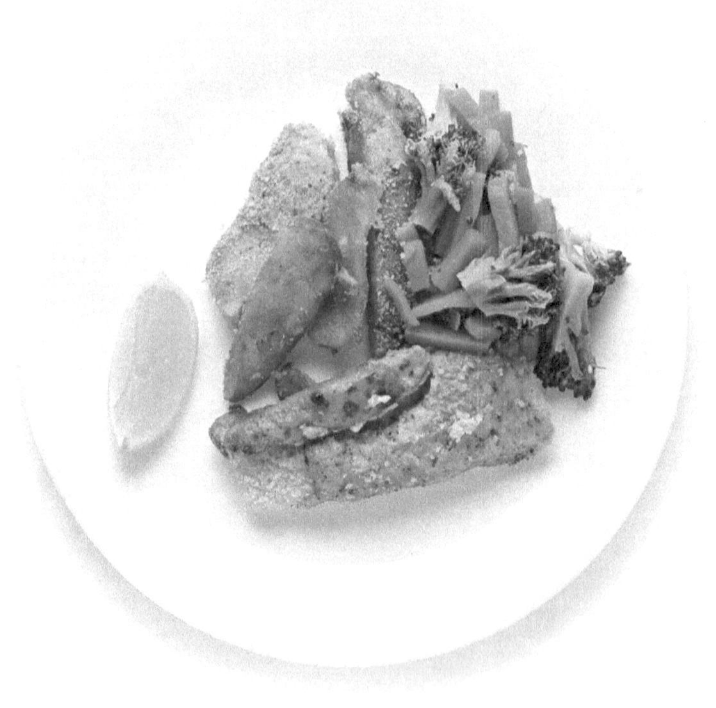

Biggest Loser
Diet

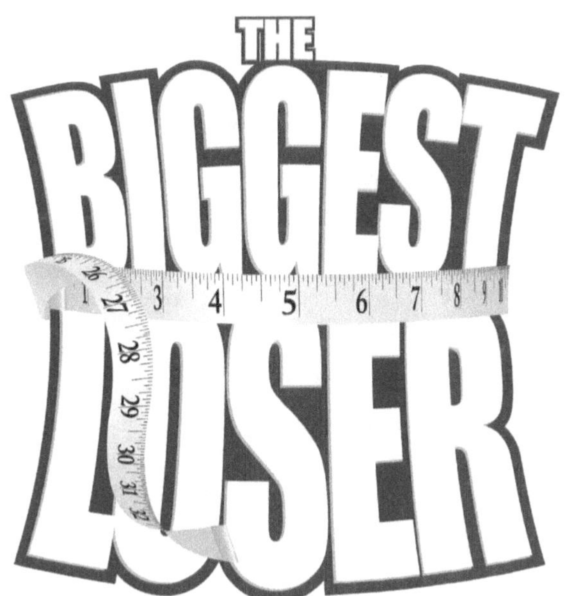

Zone Diet

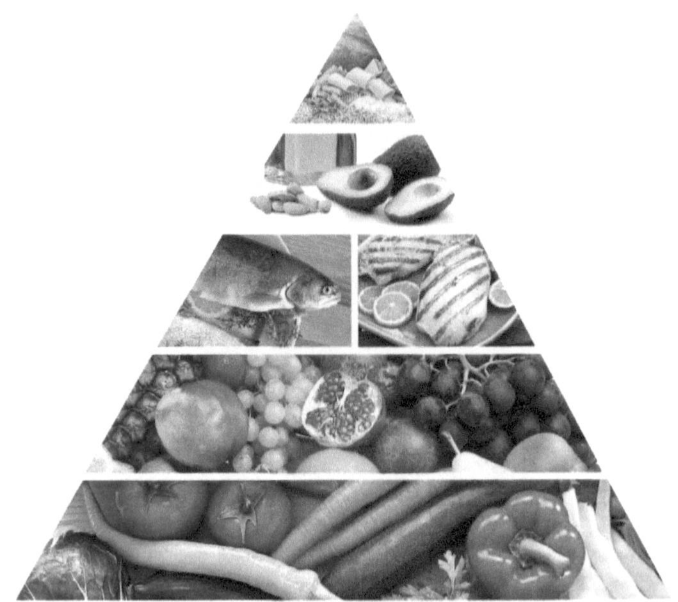

Mind Diet

Wild Diet

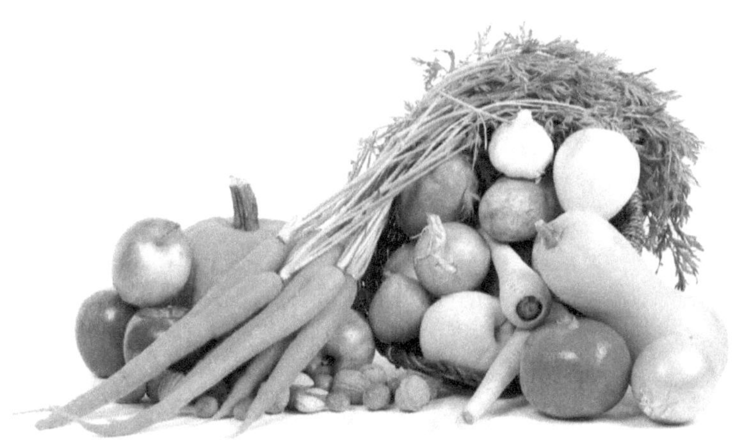

Ketogenic Diet

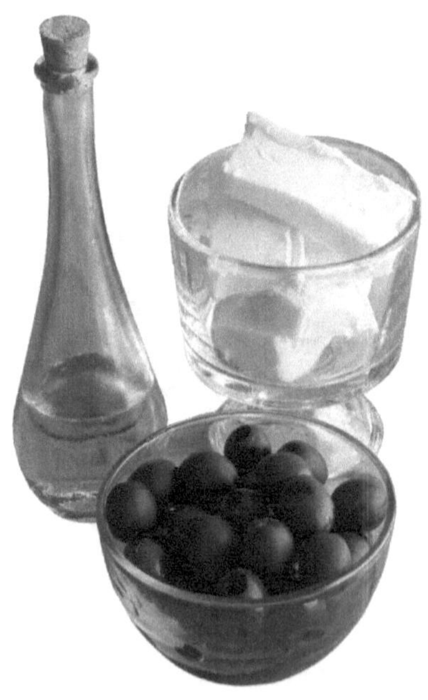

Whole30 Diet

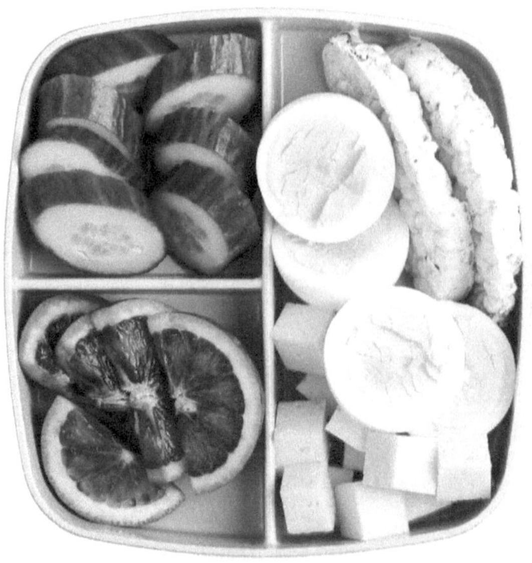

Macrobiotic Diet

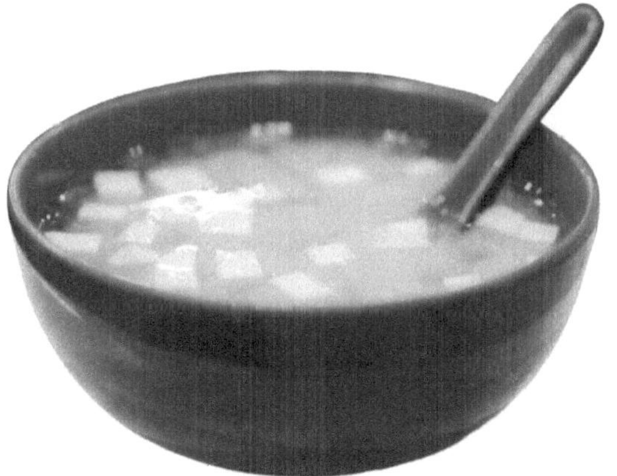

Wild Diet

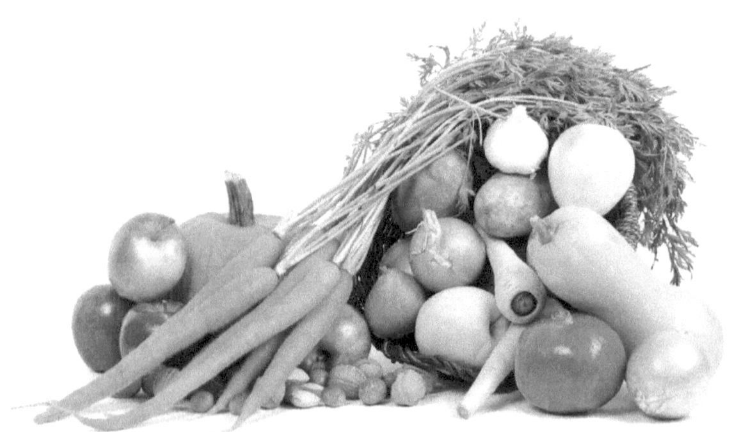

Chapter 4) Lets lose those extra pounds!

I was" thinking that if I could lose some weight I would stop feeling sharp trigger pain everywhere and my lumbar would stop getting stock each time I seat for 30 minutes." And that my friend, would be the number 1 reason to get started!!! So let's do it! It was very hard to get going, I started by walking with music along the river then I switch to nature trails so I didnt have to feel self-conscious, I then gathered nutritional journals and workout plan from multiple health sources and choose a different one every day and try to follow the steps my best way i could, I then introduced the jumping cord in my walk for a short 2 min to 3min then added zumba twice a week and yoga once a week and at home I stop eating breads after noon and ate broccoli and celery everyday, every other day after a fast walk I all have a slim fast and eggs if I work my muscles, I'll eat nuts and raisins, banana and drink only vitamin water and diet sodas. I enjoy stretching and static resistance but to really lose pounds I had to use a pedometer and stopwatch to push myself to run more, a little extra time each time and while I was at it, I would include crunches, jumps, quads and resistance exercises, after I was able to walk a good fast 20 minute I started to add a 2 minute run every 5 minute and gradually increase. What really help to boost energy was eating fish, broccoli, spinach, and dark chocolate accompanied with a slim fast to make sure I was getting all the nutritional nutrients needed, on hard days I allow myself to go to a buffet and eat all the salads and seafood, My favorite is: salmon and shrimps" I want. Once I started to feel lighter and won't feel out of breath too quickly, everything got much easier and that's how I started to increase my runs and sport activities and too make sure I wouldn't get trapt into a booring routine I try to gain new sport activities interest by trying a little of everything but skipping this intense work out and I saw the weight drop off within weeks, When you see it you don't really want to screw it all up by eating sweets and fat so your mind is too content it won't allow it by remembering how hard it was to loose. I went down to 155 but a year later I didn't keep all of it off because I was also using my workout to manage my drinking so for me! and that is just me (every weight loss journey is different) To be able to off alcohol and being healthy I had to find an in-between balance I could handle without the help of alcohol so I'm now around 175 but I know their space for improvement....

Here are some exercises you can start with you can also check out your fitness magasine and try to find a better fit for you.

Dance Fitness, Zumba, Hip Hop classes:

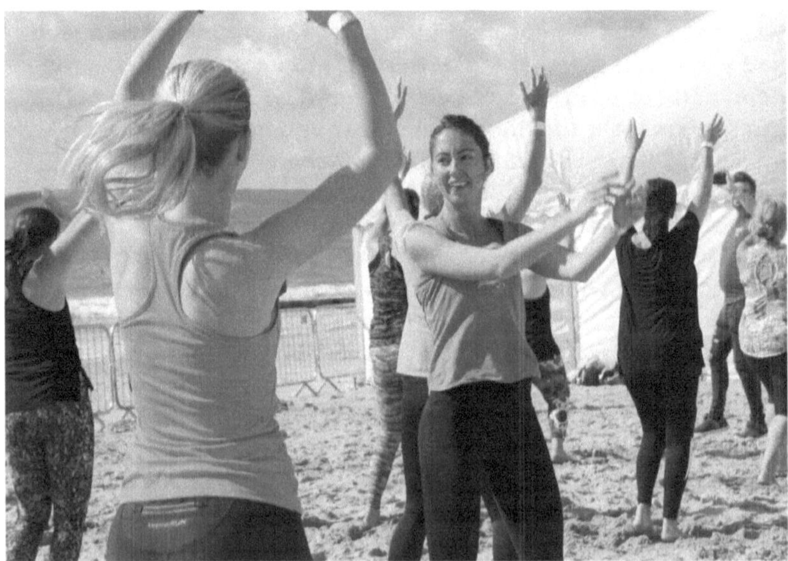

Cardio Dance: In this fun class, you will dance your "body off" with African dances, Hip hop, Rock, Twist, salsa, Rumba,

Merengue, French, bachata, Rumba, jazz, Socca, reaggaton, Dance Halls, etc. ...any dance that will make you more than happy to learn and enjoy! During this class you will challenge your cardio, strength and flexibility.

Zumba: Zumba classes are typically about an hour long and are taught by instructors licensed by Zumba Fitness. The exercises include music with fast and slow rhythms, as well as resistance training. The music comes from the following dance styles: cumbia, salsa, merengue, mambo, flamenco, chachacha, reggaeton, soca, samba, hip hop music, axé music and tango

Cardio Dance and Core: In this class we will have the workout out of a Cardio dance and we will also have the opportunity to strengthen your core. We will most likely have 15 minutes dedicated to our core.

Gentle Fitness: A gentle class that strengthen and conditioning the body by alternating cardiovascular and strength training exercises. There also dance ballroom, and other type of group dance you could be interested in, there always this free dance program video on youtube if you need a push.

Abdominal Crunch

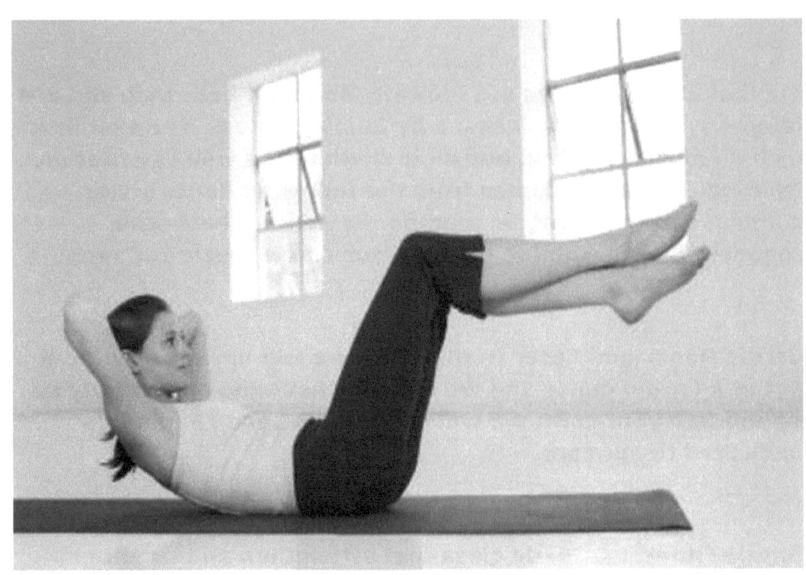

Doing Yoga Makes Me a Better Runner, but It's Got Nothing to Do With Flexibility:

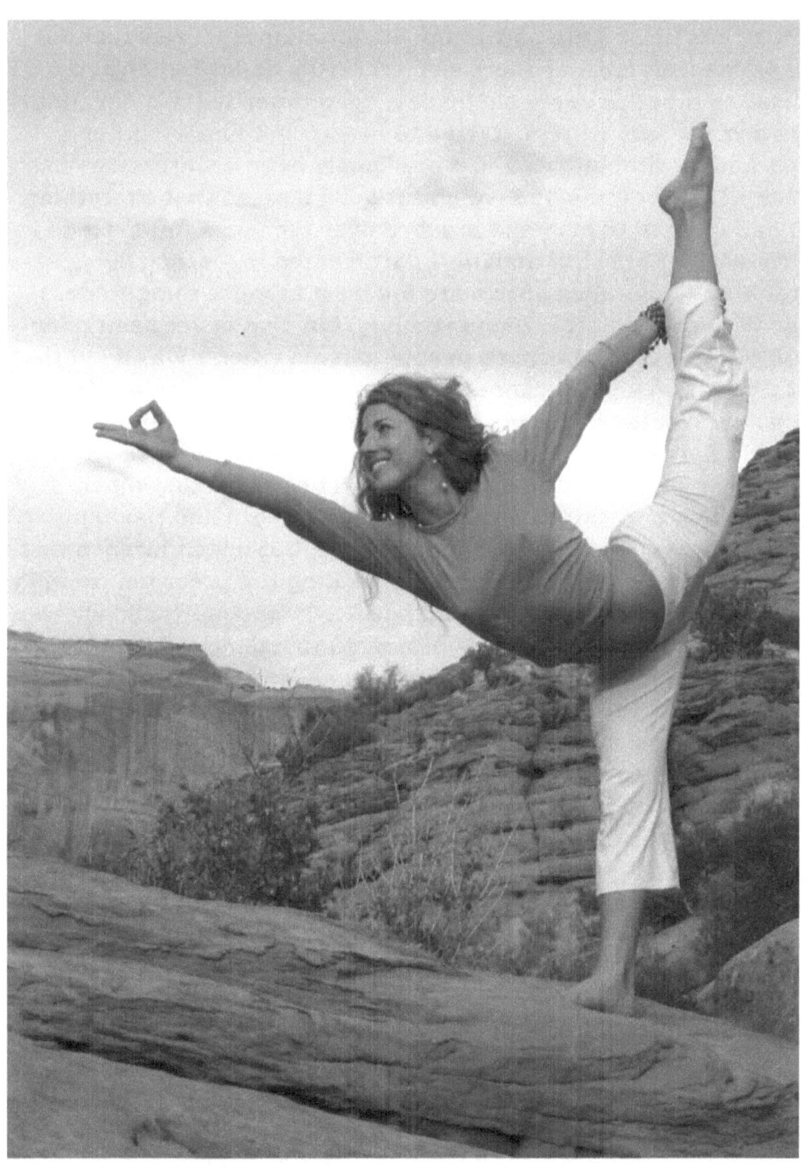

Here is a woman own word story:

Yoga has been a big part of my life for almost 10 years, and it was the first form of exercise I ever truly dedicated myself to. I used to practice every single day, sometimes twice a day, until two years ago, when I started to branch out and try other pockets of fitness that I had previously been disinterested in, like HIIT workouts and weightlifting. I noticed that everything I had learned in my yoga practice over the years influenced every other physical activity I participated in, especially running. Endurance sports are my least favorite thing to do. I don't know what it is about running, but I've never been a fan of it. Perhaps it's because people told me when I was a kid that I'd never be a great runner due to my short legs (mean, I know). Whatever the case is, you'd much sooner find me picking up a barbell than lacing up a pair of running shoes.In the past several months, though, I've been devoting much more time and energy to running. My strength and flexibility have always been in pretty good shape, but my endurance was lacking. So I religiously started attending the precision running classes at Equinox, which are specifically and methodically created to help you get better at distance running (and make you sweat buckets). My first few weeks were pretty miserable. I wasn't used to doing that kind of intense cardio for a full hour, and there were many times when I simply wanted to quit. I soon realized that running was more of a mental challenge than anything else. You have to be OK with being stuck in an uncomfortable state for an extended period of time. When I really thought about this, though, I came to see that this was the same exact principle I'd learned and sharpened in yoga. So I took the resilience and mental fortitude it takes to hold Warrior 3 for what seems like forever, and I transferred it to my running sessions. This helped me push through the toughest of courses with a steady mind. Furthermore, my yoga practice has made me acutely aware of my body, which I realize is a cliché phrase you always hear in yoga, but it's true. When I began the running classes at Equinox, I was able to take all the feedback from the running instructor and apply it right away. For example, as soon as he told me my right hip was tight, which was causing my right leg to lag behind, I immediately created a yoga sequence for myself that loosened up my right side and allowed me to even out my stride, helping me to run faster. Each time my instructor comes to me with a correction now, I feel confident that I can execute it in real time because I know how to isolate my attention to one specific part of my body . . . and it's all thanks to my yoga practice. I may never be a champion marathon runner, but the more I apply my yoga practice to running, the easier it gets and the more I can enjoy every mile. And that's all that really matters in the end.

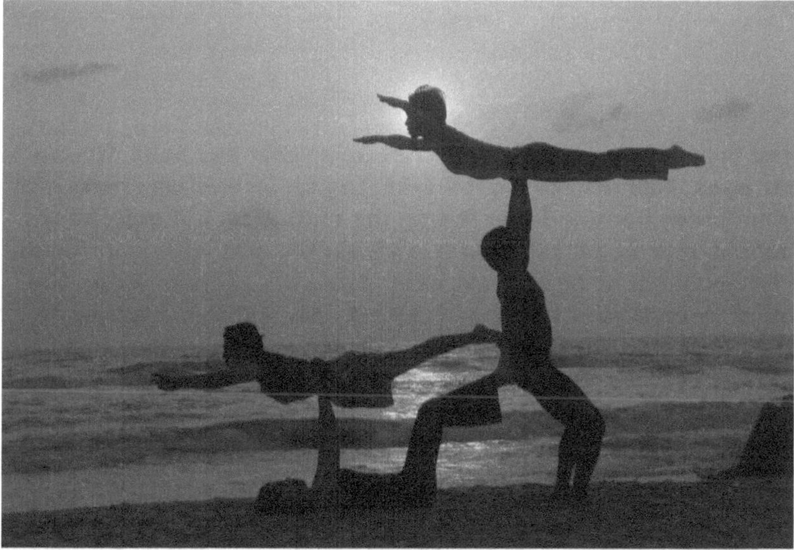

Bicycle Crunches:

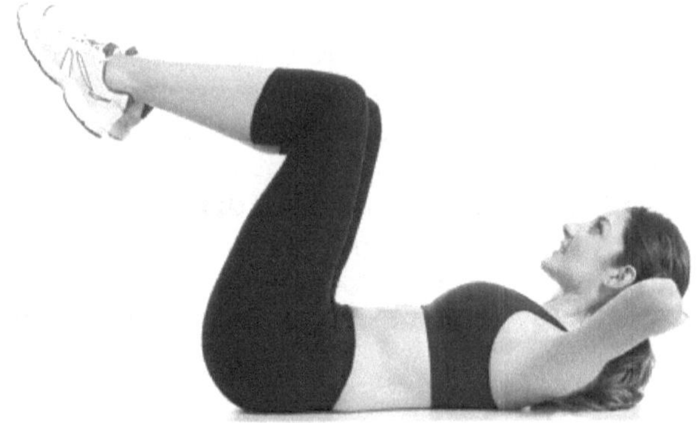

The bicycle is an old fashioned exercise that has been around for ages. This is because it works. Lay on an exercise mat, with your knees bent and feet flat on the mat. Also, put your hands behind your head. Lift your head from the mat with your hands still behind your head. Next extend one leg while bringing the other toward your chest. Touch that knee with your elbow on the other side with your hands still locked behind your head. Extend that leg back out and touch the other knee with your alternate elbow. Continue alternating legs, bringing the opposite elbow to touch the bent knee. This should resemble riding a bicycle.

Leg Lifts

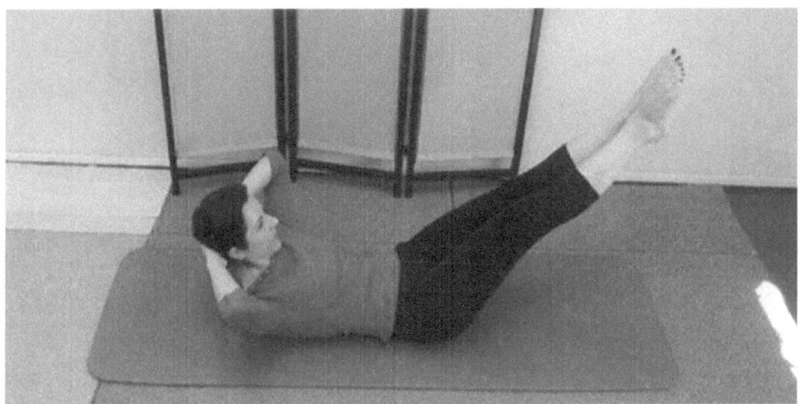

Leg lifts are perfect for strengthening the lower stomach. To do leg lifts, lay on your back with your legs extended. Lift your legs, pointing your toes to the ceiling. As slowly as you can, lower your legs to the floor. Repeat this exercise 10 times. If this is too difficult, you can do it one leg at a time. This exercise also works your butt.

Fitness Ball Crunches

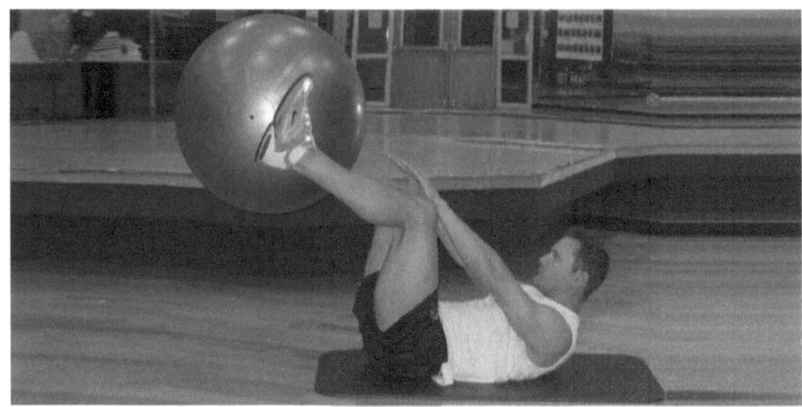

Crunches are an excellent way to strengthen the midsection and using a fitness ball makes it much easier in that it takes the pressure off your back. As you do your crunches, allow the ball to roll backwards as you crunch forward and roll forward as you move back. Muscles Targeted: A strong abdominal section is vital for maintaining good posture. Although, much attention is paid to the abs, the muscles closer to the spine are far more significant. There are three muscle groups that form the abdomen. The transverse abdominis, internal obliques and external obliques. The transverse abdominis is the closest to the spine and cannot be touched from the outside of the body. The internal obliques form each side of the torso and aid in rotational and lateral flexion of the spine. The external obliques are another pair of muscles that help with the same function as the internal obliques only to a lesser extent.

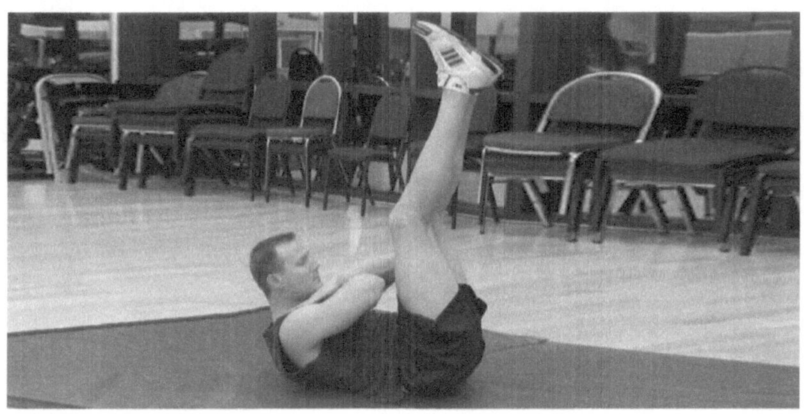

Reverse Sit-ups

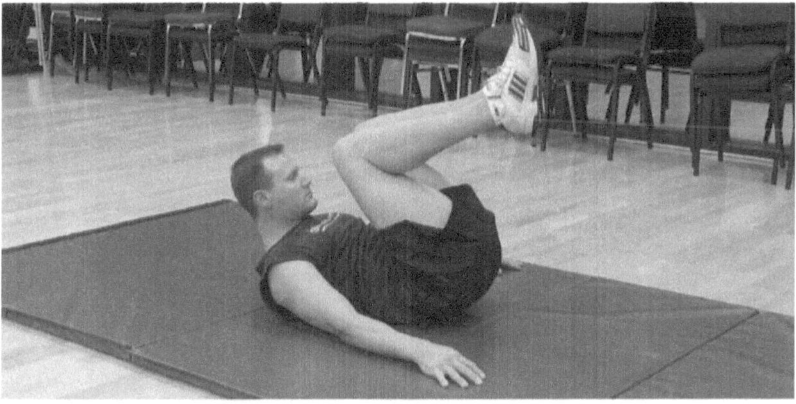

Sit on the exercise mat with your knees bent and arms out in front of you. Lay back as far as you can holding that position for as long as you can without collapsing. Repeat this exercise five times.

Stretch Your Midsection

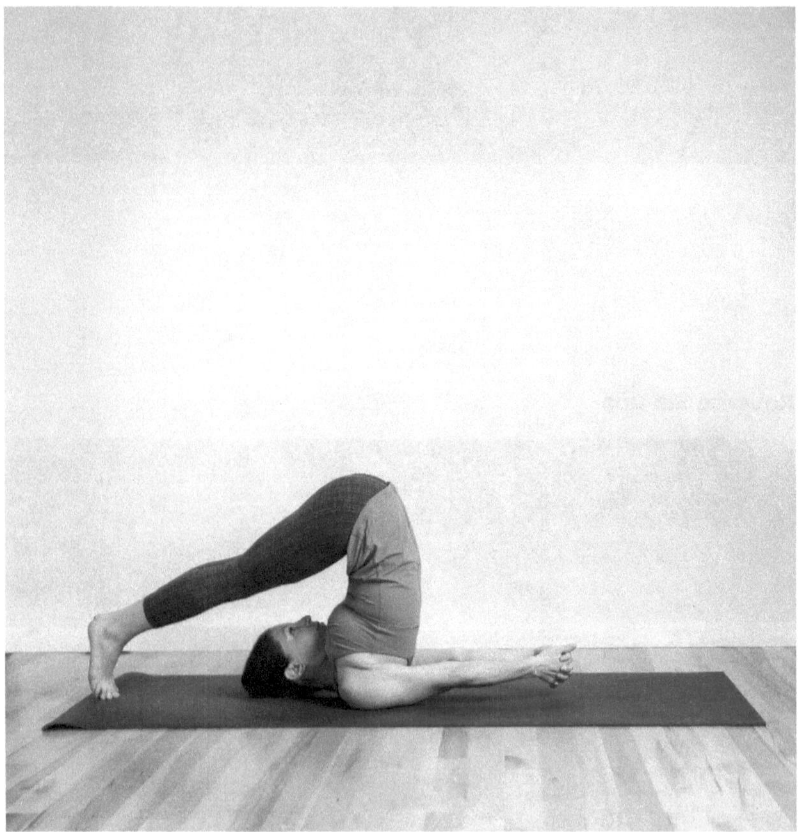

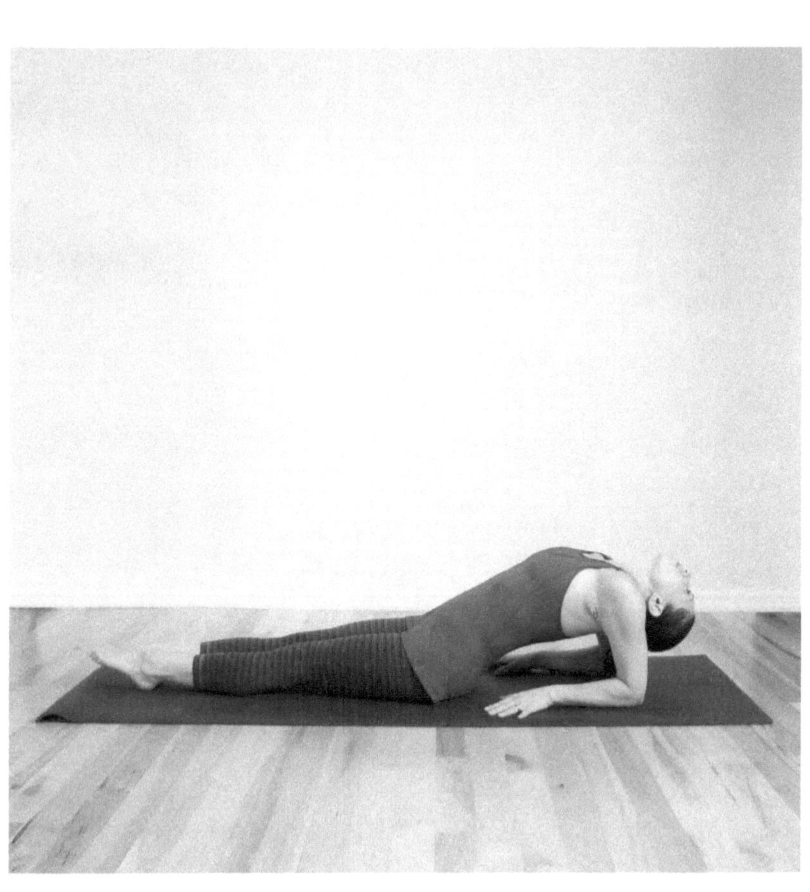

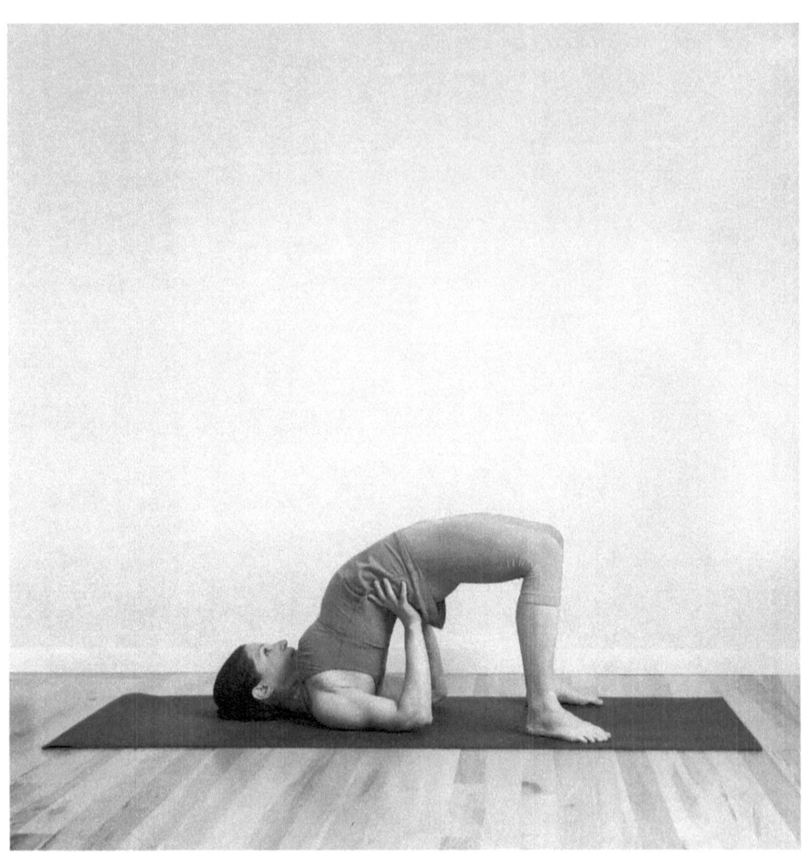

Before and after doing abdominal exercises, it is important to stretch. To stretch your abdominals, lie on the exercise mat face down in push-up position. Push up with your arms, keeping your pelvis on the floor. Next, stand up and do a whole body stretch, clasping your hands above your head and pushing your palms toward the ceiling.

Here are 3 different body type of workout woman

It's always nice to see it! so you can imagine what you body could look like even if you never come close to have that many muscles and look that sharp,you still appreciate having a nicer looking body.

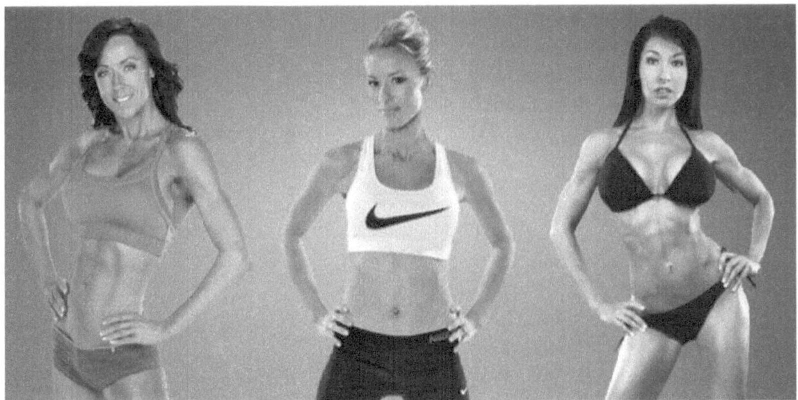

I hope you all the best for your weight loss challenge and I hope that my story will help you to continue your pursuit of a better body. Please don't gave up because it does get hard and even if you regain a little don't beat yourself up try to remember that the most valuable lesson here to lose weight easely it's to enjoy moving our body so this effort become a enjoyement instead of a chore, find that special activity who gets you going and use it in your favor.

BY Author,Vanessa Bush

Make all your wishes come true!

Lose the weight you need to lose now!

Don't wait, challenge yourself!